The First Month Guide To A Healthy Living

Volume 2

of the series

Living Positive

AMR AL-HARIRI MD

ISBN:1518610129
ISBN-13: 978-1518610127

DEDICATION

To all the parents that are doing their best to maximize the potentials of
their children

We understand what you are trying to do

CONTENTS

1   Getting Fit For Life in The First Month   1

2   Joining The Gym in The First Month   20

3   Yoga in The First Month   39

4   Vegan – The First Month   58

AMR AL-HARIRI, MD

A practicing Neurologist in California with the following board certifications:

American Board of Psychiatry and Neurology

American Board of Internal Medicine

American Board of Pediatrics

I Invest in Positive, Let it Flow into Your Life

1 GETTING FIT FOR LIFE IN THE FIRST MONTH

So, you've decided you want to be fit for life. That is a great goal because as we all know being fit for life means living a longer life.

Before we go any further, let's all be aware of one very important fact - those 3 simple words "Fit for Life" hold a boat load of changes that will have to take place over time. It will be day to day, month to month, and sometimes even minute to minute to get from your current state to being Fit for Life. However, if you do it that way, very slowly, then new habits will form and the changes will be permanent.

That's because slow change is usually permanent change. Experts say it can take up to one year to permanently change a habit. A study published in the British Journal of Health Psychology last year*, studied the formation of habit. A habit is a learned, automatic response to certain cues. To form a new habit, the scientists say it "requires the initiation of a behavior and repetition in a constant context. "

What on earth does that mean? I'll explain. As an example, let's choose a habit that we hear a lot about, that is very hard to break, that of wanting a cigarette with a cup of coffee, or after sex! The behavior is smoking and the constant context is the cup of coffee or sex. Coffee, cigarette, coffee, cigarette, repeat- repeat- repeat, and you have a habit! If you remove the coffee, a smoker might not necessarily want a cigarette in that exact time and place.

In other words- when something specific happens you have a learned, repeated response and that is a habit! What are some other common habits? Coffee and donuts. Putting your seatbelt on in the car. You get in the car, that is the context, and you reach for the seatbelt- the behavior.

There are as many habits as there are people- the habit of putting on pajamas when they get home from work, the habit of toast and coffee for breakfast, or reading before going to sleep.

In order to form a new habit, you have to have a context for that habit that occurs regularly. I know- we are getting rather scientific here but if we don't understand how to form new habits, how do we expect to?

Think about what new habit you want to form in your first month of becoming fit for life? Notice I said "Habit" singular, not "Habits" plural. We're taking it slow and steady. To talk about how to create a new habit, let's choose drinking water because it's one of the simpler habits to talk about. The British Scientists we referred to earlier found that the strength of any habit depends upon repetition, developing a new habit as part of an everyday routine and then reinforcing the habit.

When it comes to drinking more water, think about where you might connect that with part of your existing daily routine. You cannot expect to change your routine AND develop new habits. That is too much for any human being! How would you create context, or a trigger, for the new habit of drinking water?

Opportunity Number One: You probably drink coffee at home in the morning, then go to work and drink more coffee. What if when you got your coffee at work you also got a glass or bottle of water as well? That connects water with work and coffee. It places the new habit in a routine that already exists.

Opportunity Number Two: Whatever you do when you get home from work, it definitely involves drinking something. Why not just add a glass of water to that? Now you have created another opportunity for the new habit to take hold.

The point is this- whatever new habit you want to form, think about where it fits into your existing routine. Identify what activity in your existing routine can serve as a trigger for the new habit of drinking water. Once you have determined that, it's just repeat, repeat, repeat.

Let's move on. What are the first steps you need to take during the first month of your trek toward being Fit for Life? You need to get organized and then you need to select the first few things that you want to change. Not too many! It will all fall apart if you do that.

Organization is Number One. You need to organize your cupboards, your fridge and your closet.

Let's Head to the Kitchen Cupboard

Before you can make the lifestyle changes that will increase your fitness level, you have to eliminate traps, tripping mechanisms and gaping potholes in your cupboards!

- You want to head toward the fridge when you are hungry, not the cupboard. The fridge holds healthy yogurts, fruits and vegetables. The cupboard holds dangerous salty, high carb, high sugar snacks.

- Open your cupboards and remove all the fatty, sugary snacks that are tempting when you are tired and hungry. Or, just because you love them! If you live alone, put all these snacks in a bag and take them to the office. Your co-workers will love you (maybe!).

- If you live with your family, and you need to leave the snacks for them, then put the snacks in one cupboard only. Do not store them all through the kitchen. Now your job is to avoid that one cupboard. This will also prevent you from being detoured unexpectedly when you open the cereal cupboard and find cupcakes staring you in the face!

To the Fridge

Time to organize the fridge! If you live alone this will be fairly easy. If you live with your family it will be a bit more challenging. Here's how to approach it:

- All good foods should be easily accessible at the front of the shelf-

    - This is where you put dishes of fresh fruit, cut veggies, pre-cooked chicken

- If you are starving when you get home, make sure you have food to crunch on right away.

- Keep cheese sticks, small yogurt cups, grapes and other easily eaten foods in the fridge.

- Ice cream should be in the back of the freezer

- Frozen treats that you have planned for should be in the front.

And remember- your home does not have to be a democracy! If your kids, or your partner, repeatedly eat the food that is for you, fine. Don't buy the other snacks! Now the entire family is getting healthy. If they kick and scream because you stopped buying Doritos, buy them again, but your food is strictly hands off!

Easy Access to Water

None of us drink enough water. Science wavers and changes about whether we need to drink eight 8 ounce glasses of water every day. It doesn't matter. What holds true is that if you are going to get fit, and stay fit, you need to be hydrated. And that means drinking more water than you are probably drinking right now. This will only work if you have easy access to water.

- Do you like water cold? If so, either fill a pitcher every day and put in the fridge, or buy gallons of water and put them in the fridge. Place them at the front of the shelf!

- It may sound silly, but it helps to drink out of a nice glass. If you usually grab whatever is handy-sippy cup, plastic beer cup, measuring cup, you aren't going to want to drink much water! What if you kept a crystal glass in the fridge, or on top of the fridge, just for you? Now drinking water is very enjoyable and if you are always on the run, it may even feel like a brief moment of luxury.

- Keep water at your desk. This is where a glass water container-the type where the glass fits upside down on the top, comes in very handy. Fill the container and you have water for a couple of hours, and, you can drink out of a nice glass!

Let's talk about one problem. If drinking water makes you go to the bathroom all the time, it is not going to be practical at work. You can't keep getting up from your desk or leaving meetings to run to the restroom. In this case, you will have to find another solution. It might be drinking water in the early morning or when you get home from work. Or, it may mean you can only drink a lot of water on the weekends.

What is most important is this: your healthy changes have to make sense and have to be incorporated into your lifestyle or they won't stick. Remember what we have discussed about the science of forming new habits, and you will be successful in becoming fit for life.

Ok. So back to our organization.

Choose a simple workout and a simple approach to success.

Don't try to become a triathlete the first month or even the first year. Oh no. This is not the time to go whole-hog – it's one step at a time. This is the time to find activities that you love – the ones that don't feel like exercise.

Step Number One: Just like good food, your workout gear needs to be handy or you won't use it.

- If you go to the gym, put your gym bag by the door.

- If you walk, put your sneakers by the door.

- If you walk first thing in the morning, put your workout clothes by the door in your bedroom and put them on when you get up. It's much harder not to walk when you are already dressed in your walking clothes!

- If you use exercise videos at home, put them on top of the VCR.

- If you take a yoga, spinning or dance class, put it on your schedule and plan around it.

The fewer steps you have to go through to get to exercise the more successful you will be.

Organize Your Closet:

Fit for Life means being realistic. If you are a size 16 and you keep a size 8 dress in the closet as motivation to lose weight- take it out of your closet! Why? Because every day you don't fit into that dress is another day that you get discouraged. Every day that you stare at that dress and can't wear it is another day you think less of yourself. Now is the time to stop beating yourself up.

Here is what you do: Remove any clothes from your closet that are too tight or too small. It's time to establish a healthy bottom line. Start your trek to Fit for Life from a place where you feel good about yourself, wearing clothes that look good and feel good. Look at yourself in the mirror and know that those clothes will get bigger and bigger. When they do, you will have the fun of buying new clothes. But starting today, those small clothes in your closet are going to stop causing you frustration! Now is the time to stop beating yourself up. You are powerful, you are worthy, and you are strong! That is your new mantra.

Now, we have talked about how to form new habits, how to remove traps and potential sabotage in your kitchen cupboards and your fridge, and we have talked about how to set yourself up to form a new habit of exercising in some way that you love.

We have a couple more things to discuss.

The first is how to break old habits.

We talked about the science of forming new habits, but how on earth do you break the new ones?

When you stop for coffee, is there always a donut, pastry or fast food breakfast sandwich to go with it? If so, that is probably at the top of the list of very hard-to-break habits! Here is an idea of how to do it.

Number One: You can just go cold turkey and not order the donut with the coffee. This is only a good idea for adventurous types.

 Number Two:

In Week 1, instead of ordering two donuts, order just one. Better to wean yourself off the morning goodies then risk withdrawal. We prefer this easy-does-it approach. Order one a day for a week.

Week 2: Once you are down to just one donut, eat only half. Throw the rest out the window. The birds will love you. Do this for one week. Or half a week if you are getting a new rhythm.

Week 3: No donuts, just coffee. But hold on a minute-

Remember what we said about forming new habits? Behaviors become habits with repetition and with the same triggers. Time to fool your old habit of coffee and donuts. What about coffee with graham crackers and peanut butter? If you like rice cakes or popped cakes, what about those, or a banana with peanut butter? Your tasted buds will say Yum before your old habit can say "Hey wait a minute!"

The second thing we have to discuss is the mental game of getting fit.

Many days you are not going to want to participate in any activity except sitting in a chair. When you are tired you are going to want to eat your favorite ice cream. And after a hard day at work, or an argument with a loved one, cookies are going to seem like a great answer to the problem!

We are all like that. We all have our favorite crutches and it doesn't always include food. But, since we are talking about getting fit for life, food is at the core of the matter.

I'm not a psychologist, (and I don't even play one on TV!), so I'm not going to talk about the psychology of eating for comfort. Let's just say this- if you have a really bad day- and you need comfort food, go ahead and eat it. That's right- go ahead and eat it. Just don't eat it the next day and the next. The key to success is weaving the high calorie days in with the low calorie days.

Another key is weaving active days in with the inactive days. If you realistically can't move more during the week, that's ok. Don't beat yourself up about it! Decide to become more active on the weekends. Instead of sitting inside all day Saturday and Sunday, join a walking club, or a free Zumba class, or walk the beach, walk downtown, or find any number of free activities available in any community. It's not hard to do. When you start looking for new activities you are going to find there are a lot of them, and you never knew they existed!

Many communities now have rental bikes located throughout town. You don't have to live in a big city to find that. What a great way to spend a Saturday! Rent the bike, tool around town, have some lunch, and then return the bike. Perfect!

I know I said we only had a couple of things to discuss before we wrap up today, but there is one more that can't be left on the table, and that is-

The safety of working out.

Many a Weekend Warrior has ended up in the emergency room seeking the valiant performance of yesteryear! Be smart, be safe, and enjoy the journey. For a solid list of safety tips we turned to Web MD**, generally regarded as a reliable source of health information.

Here are the safety tips you need to remember:

- Start slowly. Doing too much, too soon, can hurt you, especially if you have not been active.

- Don't hold your breath! Breathe out while your muscle is working, breathe in when it relaxes. For example, if you are lifting something, breathe out as you lift; breathe in when you stop.

- If you are taking any medicines or have any illnesses that change your natural heart rate, don't use your pulse rate as a way of judging how hard you should exercise. One example of this kind of medicine is a type of blood pressure drug known as a beta blocker.

- Use a helmet for bike riding. Seems like common sense but you would be surprised how many people end up in the emergency room because they thought they didn't need simple safety equipment.

- Wear the correct footwear. You can't start walking for exercise while wearing sandals, or boots, or even kitten heels! Your calves, shins, hips and thighs need proper support if you are going to put enough energy into walking for it to help you get fit for life!

- Drink plenty of water while exercising and sweating. Stay hydrated!

- Warm up your muscles before you stretch. For example, do a little easy biking, or walking and light arm pumping first, then stretch.

- Exercises should not hurt or make you feel really tired. You might feel some soreness, a little discomfort, or a bit weary, but you should not feel pain

NOW, Ready, Set, Go and get fit for life! You are on your way! And remember, every journey begins with a single step, so take it one step at a time. We're with you!

Resources:

*Forming a flossing habit: An exploratory study of the psychological determinants of habit formation

Gaby Judah1,*, Benjamin Gardner2, Robert Aunger1 Article first published online: 18 SEP 2012, DOI: 10.1111/j.2044-8287.2012.02086.x British Journal of Health Psychology, Volume 18, Issue 2, pages 338–353, May 2013.

2 JOING THE GYM IN THE FIRST MONTH

Oh boy, whether you are joining a gym to fulfill a New Year's Resolution, on the insistence of your physician, or just because you don't like what you see in the mirror, you have made a big step toward better health. Congratulations! It's going to be fun some days, hard on others, but every day spent at the gym will take you toward good health and wellness, and that is certainly worth all the hard work!

Hopefully you conducted your due diligence before joining the gym. You know, joining a gym is a little like getting married. You financially bound to the gym of your choice and you are going to invest a lot of time in it to make the relationship work! On the other hand, the gym isn't going to get mad if you don't show up, they will just continue to take your money. In fact, your gym is more than willing to take your money whether you go five times a week or five times a year.

Just to make sure we are all on the same page when it comes to the important ABC's of joining a gym, let's briefly review the things you should check out before paying for a membership.

- **Location** - This is the single most important element in your decision. A gym can have every bell and whistle in the world, but if it's too far away, there's a good chance you won't go. Make sure the gym is either close to your house or your job.

- **Hours** - This is an obvious one, but often overlooked by many of us, assuming that most gyms are open all hours of the day. Double-check to make sure the gym is available for the times and days you want to work out.

- **Child care** - Check the hours of the child care facilities (some only operate within certain hours) and the space. Is it overcrowded? Do they have enough employees? Make sure you're comfortable leaving your kids there before you commit to a membership.

- **Cost** - Gyms operate in different ways, but you'll likely have to sign a contract and pay a certain amount each month. The nicer the gym and the nicer the membership, the more you'll pay.

- **Look for specials** - Most gyms offer monthly specials -- waiving the initiation fee, free personal training, or a few free months. Ask the salespeople about any specials available before signing on.

What about paying for classes?

Are classes included in your monthly fee, or do you have to pay an additional fee for them once you join? Do you have to pay for them ahead of time (say, six months' worth)? Does the gym offer one free class so you can find out if it's right for you?

Research - Too many people take the first offer, rather than shopping around to nearby clubs. Making the rounds to every gym in the area will give you an idea of what people are charging and the specials they're offering. That puts you in a position to negotiate an even better deal.

- **Read the fine print** - Is there a penalty for getting out of your contract early? Is there an option to put your membership on hold if you get injured, sick or have a long trip? Find out the options included in your membership before you sign up.

- **Be careful about signing a long-term contract**. While paying in advance will probably get you a better rate, most experts agree it is preferable to pay month-to-month. When you're presented with the contract, do not sign it on the spot. Resist high pressure sales techniques and stick to your guns -- don't sign anything until you've had a chance to go home or another quiet location and review it with a fine tooth comb. Even better, have someone else read over it in case they spot something you don't.

- **Features** - Make sure your gym has the activities you want to participate in -- racquetball, tennis courts, a pool, fitness classes, specific machines or equipment, personal training, physical therapy, etc. Does it offer yoga?

- **Atmosphere** - While you may not want a jam-packed gym, having people around can add energy to your workout. Pay attention to how the gym feels. Is the music too loud? Are there waiting lines for any machines? Is there enough space for people to do their workouts? Do you feel comfortable? If you're there for serious exercise and it feels like a dance club, you may not be as motivated to work out there.

- **Environment** - Is the gym clean? Is it spacious? If it's a dump, you may not be too thrilled to work out there. What about TVs? Do they have plenty around the cardio machines so you don't get bored? Can you listen to the stations on your headphones? Are there spray bottles around the gym so people can wipe down the machines? Are the bathrooms clean and well-stocked? These are the small details that can make your workouts more of a chore than they have to be.

Parking - During busy hours (often after work), make sure you don't have to spend an hour looking for a place to park.

Ask about the qualifications of the trainers

Unfortunately there is no one association that sets qualifications for trainers in gyms in the United States. Some gyms, however, do require that their trainers achieve certification from the American College of Sports Medicine, the largest sports medicine and exercise science organization in the world. Ask if the staff is certified by this organization or a similar one. A gym with qualified staff is preferable over one that does not have requirements for its staff.

First is the orientation.

Some gyms offer the services of a free personal trainer, at least during your first visit to the gym. The staff will talk to you about gym etiquette, where you locker is and other details. Then the personal trainer will meet with you. S/he may do the following, so don't be alarmed: they will take your weight and measure your body fat percentage. You won't be happy, but that is why you joined the gym! Just acknowledge that you are dissatisfied with your current shape, but give yourself credit for joining the gym to address it!

Next the personal trainer will show you how to use the basic strength training machines. Good trainers will give you some ideas for exercises and how to perform them in repetitions and sets. They will also show you how to use different cardiovascular machines.

You won't learn all the weight training techniques or cardiovascular exercise skills in one day. This is not a formal personal training session. It's an orientation. So don't be afraid to ask questions! You are the client and you are paying to learn at the gym.

Words of warning for first time gym members

It can be very easy to hurt yourself at the gym if you don't know what you are doing. These types of injuries may become chronic so you want to avoid them by being smart and conservative in your work out. Here are a few things to remember when you start to use the equipment at the gym:

- If you are using unfamiliar equipment, do not force things around when the workout part of the machine doesn't move. Look for instructions on how to properly operate the machine. If you cannot find any, ask a staff member. The chances of hurting yourself will decrease once you know how to work out properly with the equipment. It usually isn't a good idea to ask other gym members because they may be using the equipment improperly.

- Never, ever interrupt someone who is in the middle of lifting heavy weights.
- If you sign up the gym membership with your friend, go with him or her. You will find it easier to walk into the gym the first few times if you are with a supporting buddy.
- For the first times that you go to the gym, it is a good idea to choose the less busy hours, for example mid-afternoon or late evening. Most gyms are packed early in the morning and during after work hours. You will feel more at ease if you can become accustomed to the gym when there aren't a lot of people around. You will also be able to have more time with staff.
- Don't forget to pack your soap or body shampoo and a towel if the gym doesn't provide them. You will need them if you plan to take a shower at the gym after your workout. Some gyms provide basic toiletries free of charge.

Now you have completed your very first visit to the gym. Don't expect that you will have had a good workout. It may have seemed intimidating and confusing. You may have left early, before the end of your planned workout. That's ok. It's going to take some time to feel at ease in a new environment. No one is watching you, they are in your own zone. It will take some time for you to find yours. With all the planning and anticipation you put into joining the gym, the first day may seem like it was a waste of time. Don't worry, it wasn't. Give yourself credit for going! You know a little bit about each machine. And, now that you are more familiar with the gym, you next workout will be better.

If you can afford it on your next visit, it might be helpful to hire one of the gym's personal trainers to help you establish a full workout based on your goals. The trainer will teach you how to perform a workout in correct form and how to use the machines properly for your level of fitness. You will also receive advice on your diet and motivation as well!

What do I wear?

Well, unless you are going to the gym with the sole purpose of finding a date, you wear old shorts and an old t-shirt. This isn't the ski slopes in Vail or Aspen. The gym is a place where you work hard in your own zone. If you are watching other people or worrying if they are watching you, you aren't making the most of your time at the gym.

The sneakers you wear are very important for arch, leg, hip and back support. Don't skimp on sneakers. They will support you while you work out and return every dollar you spend on them. Web MD lists the following tips on how to select a good sneaker:

- **Don't make shoes multitask.** Walking shoes are stiffer; running shoes are more flexible, with extra cushioning to handle greater impact. If you do both activities, get a pair for each one.

- **Know your foot.** Sure, we've all got 10 toes and two heels, but beyond that, feet come in a variety of shapes -- and knowing your foot's particular quirks is key to selecting the right pair of shoes. Most major brands now offer a model to suit every foot type.

- One way to determine your foot's shape is to do a "wet test"--- wet your foot, step on a piece of brown paper and trace your footprint. Or just look at where your last pair of shoes shows the most wear.

  - If your footprint shows the entire sole of your foot with little to no curve on the inside -- or if your shoes show the most wear on the inside edge -- it means you have low arches or flat feet and tend toward *over-pronation* -- meaning your feet roll inward. You'll want a shoe with a motion-control feature and maximum support.

  - If the footprint shows only a portion of your forefoot and heel with a narrow connection between the two -- or if your shoes wear out mostly on the outside edge -- you have high arches and tend to under-pronate, meaning your feet roll outward. Look for a cushioned shoe with a soft midsole.

- If your footprint has a distinct curve along the inside and your shoes wear out uniformly you have a neutral arch. Look for a "stability" shoe that has the right mix of cushioning and support.

- Measure your feet twice a year. Podiatrists say it is a myth that an adult's feet don't change. They do and you can only get the right fitting sneakers for your workout if you measure your feet when you buy new footwear.

Now that you are a regular gym-goer, there are several important personal safety tips that you need to remember. Whether or not the gym told you these things during orientation you should know them and take them to heart. These tips will keep you safe and well.

Number One; Watch your weights.

When you are using free weights, either on the bench or dumbbells, set the weights down gently on the floor to avoid harming yourself, and the equipment. If you're lifting heavy weights while performing a bench press, be sure to have someone act as a spotter to avoid having the weights fall on you. When you're finished, return all plates, bars and dumbbells to their proper racks so that others don't trip and fall on them.

Number Two: Always mop up your sweat

Mopping up your perspiration is not only sanitary, it's common courtesy and it promotes safety. A puddle of sweat on the floor could easily cause a slip-and-fall injury. Most gyms provide cleaning products and towels to wipe down machines after use. You should also place a towel on any machine before you lie down on it, in order to minimize the residual perspiration.

Drink Water

It can be easy to become dehydrated while at the gym, especially when performing aerobic exercise. Bring a water bottle with you and have it nearby while you're working out. If you prefer, many gyms offer bottled water or sports drinks for sale.

Warm Up and Cool Down

Warm up before you begin your workout. Some light stretching will make your muscles limber and more flexible, which will help prevent injury. If you're performing aerobic exercise, start slowly and build up your speed. Take the time to cool down at the end of your workout by performing light stretching.

What about infection control at the gym?

That's a good question to ask. The truth is that the number one way to stop the spread of disease and infection is to wash your hands. You can use hand sanitizer or soap and water. They are both just as effective at removing germs from your hands.

The Centers for Disease Control says, and I quote; "keeping hands clean is one of the most important steps we can take to avoid getting sick and spreading germs to others. Many diseases and conditions are spread by not washing hands with soap and clean, running water" end quote. And, the CDC recommends how to properly wash your hands. Here it is:

- Wet your hands with clean, running water (warm or cold), turn off the tap, and apply soap
- Lather your hands by rubbing them together with the soap. Be sure to lather the backs of your hands, between your fingers, and under your nails.
- Scrub your hands for at least 20 seconds. Need a timer? Hum the "Happy Birthday" song from beginning to end twice.
- Rinse your hands well under clean, running water.
- Dry your hands using a clean towel or air dry them. (Did you know that germs can be transferred more easily to and from wet hands?)

And there you have it. Five simple steps to prevent catching every cough and cold from your fellow gym members. If you wash your hands well after your workout, you know you have done everything possible to stop the spread of infection and illness from other gym members to you.

Finally, how do you stay motivated to go to the gym?
Once the newness wears off it can be a drag to haul yourself out of your car and into your workout.

- Change your perspective – Think like an athlete. Think fit. Think healthy. If you need to cut out pictures from a magazine or print them from the web to help you envision the new you, go ahead. Train your mind like you are training your body.
- Set a goal – Give yourself something concrete to work toward. It won't help if you are wandering aimlessly through weeks and months of gym time with no progress to track!
- Schedule a regular workout time- Make it your workout a habit and part of your schedule. Once

your workout becomes as important as meetings, it will be much easier to follow through!

- Think fun and variety- they say variety is the spice of life and that is never truer than when you are trying to keep a workout fresh. Vary your exercises during the week, and try different things like yoga, dance, spinning or walking.

- Reach out to others for support – find friends to go to the gym with you or join a virtual club of other fitness enthusiasts.

Well, you've done it. You have joined the gym, pulled out your old t-shirts, bought yourself the right sneakers and put yourself in a good frame of mind. Congratulations. You just put yourself on the fast track to a long, healthy life!

Resources:

CDC – Center for Disease Control and Prevention:

http://www.cdc.gov/handwashing/show-me-the-science-handwashing.html#lather

eHow – Gym Safety Rules: http://www.ehow.com/list_6498463_gym-safety-rules.html

About Health:

http://exercise.about.com/od/exerciseforbeginners/a/beforeyoujoinagym.htm

http://weightloss.about.com/od/exercis1/a/aa021507a.htm

Mun Fitness Blog:

http://munfitnessblog.com/a-must-read-guide-for-first-time-gym-goer/

3 YOGA IN THE FIRST MONTH

Yoga has many health benefits so good for you if you have started practicing! Yoga can lower blood pressure and cholesterol, reduce stress and even enhance brain function and mental focus. Practicing Yoga will give you greater flexibility, better skeletal alignment and will strengthen your bones and joints. And that's not all. Yoga can contribute to weight loss. And, for all of us who are stressed beyond reason, Yoga can create a greater sense of calm by encouraging happiness and inner peace, deeper spirituality and the integration of mind and body.

 According to the Yoga Health Foundation, Yoga isn't just a physical exercise program. It is a scientific system designed to generate greater clarity and harmony in life. With a regular practice, the foundation says that individuals often notice a stronger, slimmer and more flexible body, in addition to a mentally sharper, more patient and relaxed sense of self. Who couldn't use that?

Many health and fitness programs are difficult to maintain because they are rooted in an overall negative attitude – that you need to "fix" yourself. Yoga, on the other hand, meets you exactly where you are and does not judge. By practicing Yoga you have the opportunity to improve your health with a positive, non-forceful approach. As far as I'm concerned, those are all the great reasons to choose Yoga as your daily practice! No need for jogging here!

Let's talk about the reasons to take up the practice Yoga.

I'm going to give you Top Ten.

The Yoga Alliance says that perhaps the <u>number one</u> most important reason to practice Yoga is that it reduces stress. By encouraging relaxation, Yoga helps to lower the levels of the stress hormone cortisol. Less stress can then lower blood pressure improve digestion and boost the immune system. Less stress will also ease the symptoms of anxiety, depression, fatigue, asthma and insomnia.

Number Two: Yoga can help to ease pain. Research has shown that practicing Yoga postures and meditation, or a combination of the two, can actually reduce pain for those suffering with cancer, multiple sclerosis, auto-immune diseases, hypertension, arthritis, back and neck pain, and other chronic conditions.

Some people report that even emotional pain can be eased through the practice of Yoga.

 The 3rd reason to practice Yoga is that it contributes to better breathing. Yoga teaches people to take slower, deeper breaths. This helps to improve lung function, triggers the body's relaxation response and increases the amount of oxygen available to the body.

<u>Number Four:</u> Yoga helps to improve flexibility and mobility. It allows the Yoga practitioner to increase range of motion which will then help to reduce many aches and pains. Many people can't touch their toes during their first Yoga class. Gradually, practicing Yoga enables them to use the correct muscles in their bodies. Over time, their ligaments, tendons and muscles lengthen, increasing elasticity, and making even more Yoga poses possible. As Yoga improves body alignment it creates better posture which in turn can relieve back, neck, joint and muscle problems. In one study, people improved their flexibility by up to 35% after only 8 weeks of Yoga.

<u>The 5th reason</u> to practice Yoga is that it will give you increased strength. Yoga postures use every muscle in the body, strengthening them through the various poses. This in turn relieves muscular tension. Many of the poses, such as downward dog, upward dog, and the plank pose, build upper-body strength. The standing poses, especially if you hold them for several long

breaths, build strength in your hamstrings, quadriceps, and abs. Poses that strengthen the lower back include upward dog and the chair pose.

When done right, nearly all poses build core strength in the deep abdominal muscles.

Number Six is weight management. Yoga, even in its least vigorous style of practice can aid weight control efforts by burning excess calories and reducing stress. Yoga also encourages healthy eating habits and provides a heightened sense of well-being and self-esteem. For people who are stress eaters, or eat mindlessly because they are unhappy, lowered stress and improved self-esteem will naturally help to slow those eating habits.

The 7th reason to practice Yoga is that it improves circulation and more efficiently moves oxygenated blood to the body's cells. Cells need oxygen to remain healthy and without it they begin to decay and die, so this is an extremely important benefit of practicing Yoga.

Number Eight: You should consider practicing Yoga for

its cardiovascular benefits. Even gentle Yoga practice can provide cardiovascular benefits by lowering your resting heart rate, increasing endurance and improving oxygen uptake during exercise.

Number Nine: Yoga will help you to focus on the present. Why is that important? Because constantly living in the past or worrying about the future creates enormous stress and worry. Yoga will help you to create improved mind- body health. And it opens the way to improved concentration, coordination, reaction time and memory.

The tenth reason to practice Yoga is the wonderful benefit of gaining inner peace. The meditative aspects of Yoga help many people to reach a deeper, more spiritual and more satisfying place in their lives. Many people say that inner peace is the key reason why Yoga is an essential part of their daily lives.

Are you beginning to think that practicing Yoga is a good idea? Great!

Now let's talk about how you get ready to practice.

First, Get Geared Up- Yoga doesn't require too much equipment, but there are a few things you'll want to gather ahead of time. First and foremost is a Yoga mat. If you are beginning to practice Yoga at home, you may also want to have a Yoga block, a strap, and a blanket handy. All of these are readily available in many stores ranging from specialty Yoga stores to "big box" stores like K-Mart and Wal Mart.

Next, Get to Know Your Daily Stretches- A daily stretch routine will be the backbone of your Yoga practice, especially if you begin at home. This sequence can be done in 10-15 minutes and is designed to wake up the spine, relieve minor back pain, and stretch the hamstrings. Doing these stretches in the morning is a great way to get your day going. You can find a daily Yoga stretch routine in many websites, videos and books.

Joyce Diaz is a Yoga consultant who writes extensively on the subject. She understands that even though you have decided to begin practicing Yoga, and have decided to join a Yoga class, you may feel anxious about your first day, and you may feel intimidated when you walk into the class. As a result, she has put together 10 tips for preparing for your first Yoga class. These simple steps will help you to feel relaxed as you enter the class because you will know what to expect.

First and foremost, when you begin make sure to adjust your Yoga practice to fit your body and your level of physical fitness. Take it easy, relax and enjoy yourself. Remember, this is not an exercise class to "fix" what is wrong with you. This is a practice to achieve inner peace and spiritual, emotional and physical balance.

If you have gone over a few basic positions at home, you may feel more comfortable in class. There are hundreds of Yoga poses and your body may be upset if you select one that does not suit it, so choose the most basic Yoga posture and practice it at home. You can find these basic poses in books, videos, online, and even on television services like On Demand.

Pick a Yoga studio convenient to your home for the

sake of convenience. Getting to class should be easy, not stressful. Check the web to find a Yoga class in your neighborhood. You can also check out local gyms. Many of them offer Yoga classes.

Eat light or low-acid food before yoga, Keep things light and simple on the day of your first Yoga class. Eat something healthy at least two and half hours before class. Do not eat saucy, fried, fatty, spicy, or high-acid food before class because they take longer to digest. Just as it's a bad idea to start practice with a heavy stomach, it is also a bad idea to start on an empty stomach. You may start feeling lightheaded as the body needs fuel that is not there. If you want to eat a quick snack before class grab yogurt, fruit or vegetables. A lightly filled stomach will provide you a better practice.

Drink plenty of water before and after the class: It is very important to stay hydrated during class. This is because in a typical Yoga class you will lose water weight. Start drinking water at least two hours before your class. Your body needs time to absorb the water properly for hydration. Make sure that you're fully hydrated before you start, especially if you're doing hot Yoga. Over time, you'll learn how much water your body needs before and after class.

Wear comfortable clothes that don't restrict your movement: You don't *need* to wear long pants or spandex, just wear something you feel relaxed and confident in. Ladies may it most comfortable to wear quick-dry Capri pants and tight tops and men most usually wear shorts and baggy t-shirts. Try to avoid wearing clothes that are too loose. You don't want your top to fall down over your head while you are doing the Down Dog pose! You won't be able to see, and your classmates will be able to see more of you than you like. Remember that unlike running or other gym exercises, you will be bending and stretching a lot, so loose clothes tend to fall in your face!

Yoga is practiced barefoot: shoes and socks are generally not permitted. Being barefoot allows more grip on the mat in various poses. If you have any problem being barefoot, ask your instructor if you can keep your socks on—or invest in a pair of Yoga socks.

Get to class at least 15 minutes early: Arriving early the first day will give you enough time to fill out any paperwork that is required, put your belongings in a locker if available, and begin to relax before class. You will have time to set your Yoga mat in the room and get comfortable in the classroom. You will be able to listen to the teacher's instructions given to beginners at the beginning of the class. If for some reason you are late, be respectful of your fellow classmates and place your mat down gently so you don't disturb the class. The teacher will help you because after all, this is meant to be a calming experience, not a stressful one.

Have a brief conversation with the teacher before the class starts: Introduce yourself to the teacher. Yoga teachers are very helpful and encouraging—they want new students to have the best experience possible during their first class. And believe me, these teachers will provide adjustments and more detailed instructions if you tell them you're new. Make sure to let your teacher know of any limitations and medical conditions you have that might affect your practice. Your teacher will offer modifications where appropriate because most Yoga poses can be adjusted to your needs.

Keep your cell phones off and mind your manners: Seriously. Yoga class is not for fooling around or joking with your friends. It is not a time to keep up with phone calls, text messages or Tweets. It is a time to be quiet and mindful of your body.

So turn off your phone. If you can't live without it for one hour, then you probably aren't ready to find a quiet space within your mind.

Don't let your ego guide you: If you are practicing in a place where you feel you are being judged, then you are not in the right studio. It doesn't matter if your body isn't extremely flexible and you can't yet complete a specific pose. Always listen to your body—don't push or overextend just to keep up with the rest of the class. If the class gets to be too much for you, spend some time in child's pose (one of the first poses you will learn) until you are ready to jump back in to the class.

Thank you to Joyce for these great Ten Tips. I think that by following these suggestions, anyone can feel prepared and relaxed for their first class.

Now let's take some time to examine exactly what Yoga is, and why it is so deeply beneficial.

The classical techniques of Yoga date back more than 5,000 years. The word Yoga means "to join or yoke together". Yoga brings the body and mind together into one harmonious experience.

The system of Yoga is built on three main structures: exercise, breathing, and meditation. The exercises of Yoga are designed to put pressure on the glandular systems of the body to increase its efficiency and overall health.

In the Yoga practice, the body is looked upon as the primary instrument that enables us to work and evolve in the world, so a Yoga student treats it with great care and respect.

Yoga breathing techniques are based on the concept that breath is the source of life in the body. As you progress through the study of Yoga, you will gently increase your breath control to improve the health and function of both body and mind.

There are many types of Yoga

There are over one hundred different schools of Yoga. Each is based on a slightly different philosophy and approach to the basic practice of Yoga. It really doesn't matter which you practice. It's just interesting to know the origins of such an immensely important approach to mind-body wellness. Here are some of the most well-known.

Hatha Yoga: This is what most people associate with Yoga practice. It is the physical movements and postures of Yoga, plus breathing techniques.

Raja Yoga: This type of Yoga is called the "royal road," because it incorporates exercise and breathing practice with meditation and study.

Jnana Yoga: This Yoga is known as the path of wisdom

and is considered the most difficult path.

Bhakti Yoga: This Yoga practice is based on a practice of extreme devotion that is describe as, and I quote "one-pointed concentration upon one's concept of God" end quote.

Karma Yoga: This Yoga practice is based on the philosophy that all work of any kind is done with the mind centered on a personal concept of God.

History of Yoga

No one knows the exact year, but the practice of Yoga certainly predates written history. Stone carvings depicting figures in Yoga positions have been found in archeological sites in the Indus Valley dating back 5,000 years or more.

The tradition of Yoga has always been passed on through oral teaching and practical demonstration, one-on-one, teacher to student. The practice we know as Yoga today is based on the collective experiences of many individuals over many thousands of years.

Yoga probably arrived in the United States in the late 1800s, but it did not become widely known until the

1960s. You might have visions of Woodstock in your head when you think of the 1960's and Yoga, and that wouldn't be far from the truth. As the Youth Culture of the 1960's grew, they adopted Eastern practices and beliefs, and Yoga was certainly part of that.

As more became known about the beneficial effects of Yoga, it gained acceptance and respect as a valuable method for helping to manage stress and improve health and well-being. Many physicians now recommend Yoga practice to patients at risk for heart disease, as well as those with back pain, arthritis, depression and other chronic conditions.

What about the question of whether Yoga is a religion? Simply put, no, it is not a religion. Yoga has no creed or fixed set of beliefs, nor is there a prescribed godlike figure to be worshipped in a particular manner. The core of Yoga's philosophy is that everything is supplied from within the individual. So, there is no dependence on an external figure, either a person or a god and there is no religious organization.

Who Can Practice Yoga?

Anyone! Yoga is suitable for most adults of any age or physical condition. It is not a strenuous practice, and is an easy approach to exercise. So even those with physical limitations can find a beneficial routine of Yoga.

Can Children Practice Yoga?

Many Yoga teachers say that the exercises are not recommended for children under 16 because their bodies' nervous and glandular systems are still growing, and the effect of Yoga exercises on these systems may interfere with natural growth. However, there are an increasing number of children's Yoga classes being offered. As a parent, it is probably best that you conduct your own research on the matter and then you're your own decision. Also talk to the Yoga teacher, find out if he or she is a parent, and ask about their training and credentials.

Certainly children can safely practice meditation and simple breathing exercises as long as the breath is never held. These techniques can help children learn to relax, concentrate, and learn to reduce impulsiveness. Children trained in these techniques are better able to manage emotional upsets and cope with stressful events.

So you see, Yoga is an amazing practice that creates strength and balance, reduces stress and anxiety, and helps people of any age, from children to the elderly, to find quiet and peace in their lives.

I can't think of another type of exercise that offers that to people of all ages and physical ability.

If you have already started a Yoga practice or joined a class, congratulations! It will most likely become your lifelong practice.

If you haven't yet begun Yoga give it due consideration. It certainly is an easy way to find a calmer, more peaceful life.

Resources:

"http://**www.yogahealthfoundation.org**/images/uploads/documents/YM_10Reasons.pdf"
"http://**yoga.about.com**/od/beginningyoga/a/30dayquickstartdayone.htm"http://

"http://**yoganonymous.com**/10-tips-for-your-first-yoga-class/"
"http://**americanyogaassociation.org**/general.html"
"http://**www.webmd.com**/balance/guide/the-health-benefits-of-yoga"

4 VEGAN – THE FIRST MONTH

But first, a disclaimer. We are not here to prove or disprove the benefits of becoming a Vegan. We are here to explore it objectively and discuss what it means in terms of diet and lifestyle.

So let's begin by defining what a Vegan is. There is a difference between being a Vegan and being a Vegetarian.

A vegan eliminates all animal products from his or her diet, including dairy. Those following a vegan lifestyle generally do not wear leather and avoid products made from animals such as wool, silk and down. Vegans' humanity for animals is an abiding, overriding conviction in their lives.

Vegetarians do not eat meat, fish or poultry, but might eat dairy products such as cheese, eggs, yogurt or milk.

- Lacto-vegetarians will eat dairy, but not eggs.
- Ovo-vegetarians will eat eggs, but not dairy.
- Lacto-ovo vegetarians will eat eggs and dairy products.

The reasons for these choices are varied and based on individual beliefs. In some cases they are based on moral choices, and in others on dietary needs or simple preferences.

According to online sources, including happy cow and vegan kit, a vegan is self-committed to upholding a personal standard of living where animals are concerned. The vegan will often go beyond eliminating meat, dairy and animal products, to become an activist for animal rights. Generally, the vegan point of view is that animals are not here to be exploited by man, and that commercialization of animals involves a fundamental, inhumane component and lack of respect for basic life. A Vegan believes that cruel methods are often cheaper, and animals raised for meat or dairy products by commercial interests are commonly and routinely kept in abusive conditions and slaughtered inhumanely in the interest of a competitive marketplace. Both Vegans and Vegetarians will cite humanitarian issues associated with their choices. For example, if land used for grazing cattle was instead used to raise crops, they believe that world hunger could be easily eliminated.

Vegan Kit dot com says this: "Choosing vegan is conscientiously choosing compassion over killing, ecological preservation over destruction, health over disease, and simplicity over complexity. Each decision we make affects not only ourselves, but that of our neighbors, the planet, and all the creatures that share our earth home."

That summarizes the beliefs that lead Vegans to choose that lifestyle. Now let's talk about what being a vegan is like nutritionally and what foods the vegan diet does and does not include.

Vegan Kit says that the key to a nutritionally sound vegan diet is variety. A healthy vegan diet must include fruits, vegetables, plenty of leafy greens, whole grain products, nuts, seeds, and legumes. When you become a Vegan, you will need to work on limiting, or avoiding all together, any processed foods. They are hard to digest and I think we can all agree, vegan or not, that processed foods do not have the energy of live whole foods that are eaten the way they grow. Vegans also should eat unrefined oils like hemp, flax, coconut, and other vitamins to ensure they are eating a healthy, balanced Vegan diet.

NUTRITION

If you are not a Vegan or Vegetarian, you may believe that by virtue of the fact that they are eating lots of fruits and vegetables, their diets are always balanced. Not true. Vegan Kit tells its readers that like any diet, a vegan diet can be complete and balanced, or incomplete and unbalanced. They say that vegan eating is not a guarantee of good health. That will come as a surprise to those of us who do not eat that way. Wisely, Vegans are advised to pay attention to their food choices, watch portion sizes, limit junk and processed foods, and ensure adequate intake of a few nutrients not easily available from vegan foods. Basically, that is good advice for all of us. If we all watched our food choices, paid close attention to smaller serving sizes and limited the junk food we ate, we would be so much healthier!

The biggest question that many ask about the Vegan and Vegetarian lifestyle is, how do you get enough protein?

Come to find out, that is a great questions because the process of converting from a typical diet to the vegan diet is mostly about shifting protein sources. Doing so is not as difficult as one would think. Vegan sources say that any reasonable diet that provides sufficient calories and variety is almost guaranteed to supply enough quality protein for an average healthy vegan.

Here are the general guidelines for protein intake, based on information presented by Happy Cow and Vegan Kit. By the way, I am frequently quoting these sources because I want you to know who is giving this advice and where it is coming from. I am not a Vegan, so I cannot speak personally to this. And, it is also important that if you are interested in pursuing a Vegan or Vegetarian lifestyle, you know where to find the information.

Back to the protein issue and the recommendations from Vegan Kit:

Protein requirements will differ for each person based on age, gender, body size, physical activity, and health status. A typical vegan woman who weighs 130 pounds will need 40 to-55 grams protein each day. A typical vegan man who weighs 160 pounds will need 50 to 65 grams of protein each day.

Ok, so where do you get all those grams of protein if you are not eating meat, fish or poultry?

Well, vegans will tell you that it is actually quite easy to find protein in non-meat sources. Here is the list- get your pens and pencils ready!

Vegan protein sources include:

- soy foods including soya beans
- processed soy like tofu and soymilk
- processed soy foods like veggie burgers, hot dogs and sausage
- non-soy beans including lentils, black beans, and chick peas
- nuts and seeds
- whole grains
- mildly processed foods: like tempeh and seitan (pronounced sa-tan with emphasis on the first syllable- opposite from the pronunciation for the name of the devil!).

- Seitan is a high-protein vegetarian food made from cooked wheat gluten.

- Even vegetables will contribute 10- 20% of the daily protein requirement.

Soy can be eaten in its natural state or it can be processed. Carefully research the soy issue so that you are clear on your choices in that food category.
Soy is also a common source of food allergies and sensitivities. Anyone who appears to have ANY reaction to soy foods including rashes, hives, itching, digestive

challenges, or even breathing difficulties should stop eating soy and be evaluated by a physician.

When it comes to non-soy sources of protein, there is a long list.

It includes at least a dozen commonly available beans. Here is a partial list of them:

Pinto, black, kidney, red, navy, black-eyed peas, chick peas, yellow and green split peas, lentils, Great Northern, and Lima beans. The variety is endless and this is far from a complete list. Additional varieties of beans including cranberry, cannellini, French lentils, red lentils, and more. These beans are easily found in gourmet, organic and natural food markets.

If you don't have allergies or sensitivities to beans, then as a vegan you should be eating them at least once daily. If you're not accustomed to eating beans or you're concerned about digestive upsets or gas, start with small portions of lentils and split peas. Then slowly increase the portion size and variety of the beans you are eating.

If you do this slowly over time, you should have no problems eating beans daily.

Earlier I mentioned Seitan as a source of protein. What on earth is Seitan?

Seitan is a wheat protein that has been concentrated and separated from the naturally occurring wheat starch and fiber. It is usually sold in rolls or large pieces. Although it is very high in protein, it has no fiber. Eating Seitan is not a good idea for anyone with a wheat allergy.

Nuts and seeds are also an important and nutritious protein source. They are also a good source of healthy fats, minerals and vitamin E. Peanuts, almonds, cashews, walnuts, pumpkin seeds, sunflower seeds, flax seeds and hemp seeds are all good sources of protein. For a vegan or vegetarian, eating some type of nut, nut butter or seed every day is a good idea, and part of a healthy, balanced diet.

Now we come to the discussion of whole grains, vegetables and fruits.

As a vegan or vegetarian, you should eat mostly whole grains, such as whole wheat bread or pasta, barley, quinoa (keen-wah) and brown rice. Although white, processed grains have just as much protein as the whole-grain versions, the whole grains also provide essential B vitamins, iron, fiber and anti-oxidants. These nutrients are only found in the healthy brown layers that are removed to make grains white. White grains are fortified with some of the vitamins and iron they have lost in processing, but have no fiber or anti-oxidants. Kind of begs the question, why strip them off in the first place if you just have to put them back in?

The best way to find a healthy balance of fruits and vegetables for your diet, and this is true whether or not you are a vegan or vegetarian, is to eat as much color variety as possible; especially deep dark colors like Kale and Chard. Vegetables with deep dark colors almost always have more healthy plant chemicals than paler vegetables. It has been proven time and again that these vegetables improve heart health, contain antioxidants that help to fight cancer, and help to prevent diabetes and other illnesses. Everyone can benefit from eating a variety of colors of fruits and vegetables every day.

The most critical group of vegetables for vegans is referred to as D-G-L-V, or dark green leafy vegetables. As a group, these veggies are excellent sources of calcium, iron and scores of other nutrients. At a minimum, everyone should be eating at least three to five servings of vegetables every day, and that includes you and your family!

So, you may be thinking, "Ok, all this is great, but I still have no idea where to begin in order to eat like a vegan. Vegan Kit presents the following as an example of a typical balanced meal for lunch or dinner:

- 1/2 cup of tofu or other soy food; OR 1 cup of beans
- 1 cup of whole grain pasta, OR one cup of brown rice, OR one three-inch redskin potato
- 3/4 cup to 1 cup EACH of broccoli and carrots OR ¾ cup to 1 cup of carrots, and 2 cups mixed green salad

You should eat two to three servings of fruit each day, and fruit juice should be limited to one 8 ounce serving each day.

Now let's talk about the basic important nutritional elements that everyone, vegan or not, should have in their diet. Specifically, how does a vegan include these to ensure a healthy, balanced diet?

First, let's talk about fats and oils.

There is a lot of misinformation about the importance of fats and oils in our diet. We all need some oil every day. Without it our hair would fall out and our skin would be rough as a board. Understanding which oils are good for us is the important thing to know.

Vegan Kit says that a healthy vegan will avoid or reduce their use of foods which are deep fried or heavily coated in oil. So should the rest of us! Many of the tofu and soy meat items in Asian restaurants are deep-fried, as are many appetizers, such as egg rolls and Indian samosas. While eating deep fried foods isn't the best way to get oil into your diet, fat is essential in the diet. It also contributes to food flavor and appeal. The best guideline on how much fat and oil to include in your diet is to consider that it should comprise about 15-20% of your daily caloric intake.

The type of fat you eat matters just as much as the amount you eat. Vegans should be focusing their fat choices on olive and canola oils, avocados, nuts and seeds, nut butters, and olives.

Another important type of oil is omega-3 fats, which promote good heart health, brain function, skin health and joint health. People not following a vegan diet get their Omega-3 fats from fish. Vegans can find one type of Omega-3 fats in flax, walnuts and hemp seeds. Most vegan sources agree that a vegan DHA supplement, derived from algae, is probably a good idea, along with regular use of ground flax, hemp seeds, or walnuts.

Ok, let's move on to CALCIUM Some are concerned that a diet devoid of dairy, like that of a vegan, will also be a diet devoid of calcium. If there is no milk, cheese or yogurt in a vegan diet, where is a vegan supposed to get calcium, so important to strong teeth, bones and other organs and body functions? The answer is from plants. Not plants like trees, plants like the dark, green, leafy vegetables mentioned previously. Greens like collards, kale and turnip greens have massive amounts of important vitamins and minerals. They are some of the super foods. In fact, one cup of cooked collard greens may contain more usable calcium than one cup of cows' milk. Other calcium sources include fortified foods, such as soy milk and orange juice, almonds, figs and beans.

IRON- I think we would all agree that the majority of us, especially women, don't get enough iron.

That holds true in the statistics that show that rates of anemia among vegans are similar to that in the general population. The best vegan sources are beans and those dark, green, leafy vegetables that we keep talking about. For optimum absorption, it is recommended that vegans eat iron rich food with a source of vitamin C. For example- beans with tomatoes. Fresh spinach with strawberries. Lentils and broccoli. All those combinations sound great!

There are three other important nutrients for all of us, including vegans. They are VITAMIN D, B-12 AND IODINE.

Vegans need to pay attention to make sure they get enough of these in their diet.

Vegan sources for these nutrients are limited to fortified foods, sun-exposed mushrooms, and supplements. Vegans who decide to supplement will want to look for ergo-calci-ferol as the main ingredient.

So, we have covered a lot of territory when it comes to becoming a vegan. It is certainly a healthy way of living. In fact, I think that all of us would probably benefit from following these basic healthy guidelines, and then adding meat, fish, poultry and dairy if that is your diet preference. Eating fruits and vegetables and making sure you get enough of the essential nutrients is a cornerstone of everyone's good health.

Are there other dietary concerns that the new vegan should be aware of? Yes, a few.

The first one is that, like most Americans, vegans should be cautious about how much sodium and sugar they eat.

Vegans would be wise to target a maximum of 1500 milligrams of sodium a day and minimize their consumption of food and drinks with added sugars.

The second one concerns eating an all raw diet.

Many vegans are trying to eat an all- or nearly-all-raw diet because of increased interest in fruits and vegetables. Vegan Kit and Happy Cow say that while eating more of these foods is certainly a good idea for everyone, there are also concerns. Cooking actually liberates some nutrients in plants, and also helps to break down tough plant fibers and bitter compounds, making vegetables more nutritious and appealing. In some cases, eating the plant raw won't give you as much nutrition as if you cooked it. Also, eating a large volume of low-calorie, low protein food might support healthy weight loss, but it might also lead to unplanned, undesirable losses in weight, loss of strength, and bone density. Vegans should find a suitable balance between cooked and uncooked food. The recommendation is that uncooked food should make up approximately 1/3 of their calories, but no more than that. The rest should be cooked foods.

There are a few other considerations when you decide to become a vegan, and they are not food related. They are social concerns.

<u>Not all families are supportive of a vegan life.</u>
A family can be hesitant, or downright upset, when a loved tells them they have become a vegan. Usually this is because the family doesn't know what being a vegan is, or, they only know the commonly held myths about being a vegan. A family's reaction may be automatic and not well thought out. It may be an emotional reaction involving disappointment that you will no longer be

eating turkey on Thanksgiving or other traditional family foods. That is a strong emotional response that includes many factors and subconscious family ties.

They may even make the leap that this means that as a vegan, you will no longer be able to fully participate in family holidays.

There are as many family dynamics as there are people. Let's just say this. If your family is important to you, don't be militant about your newfound veganism.

The best thing to do is to help your family. Ease them out of their resistance by teaching them as much as you can about the vegan way of life. Help them to understand not only your philosophy, but your dedication to a healthy balanced diet that is full of all the nutrients that your body needs. Educate them about this and help them to make sure that they too are receiving the healthy nutrients they need. Try making some of the traditional family dishes in a vegan way. You need to show them that you are still able to partake in family traditions, and more importantly, that you still respect those traditions. It may take a while for your family to adapt to the fact that you are a vegan. Be as respectful as possible. After all, if you want them to respect your choices, you must respect theirs.

Above all, remember this. Your choice to become a vegan was based in part on your desire to live a balanced life. Helping your family to embrace your choices is part of that balance.

Researchers struggle to figure out how many vegans there are in the United States, but they know there are least 1 million. So if you have decided to become a vegan, you have lots of company. There are many good websites to use as well as blogs and social media sites dedicated to veganism. Educate yourself, eat well, and good luck in your new journey. Good health to you!

Resources:

http://**vegankit.com**/be

http://**www.happycow.ne**t/vegan_nutrition101.html

http://**www.wisegeek.org**/what-is-the-difference-between-a-vegan-and-a-vegetarian.htm

AMR AL-HARIRI, MD

A practicing Neurologist in California with the following board certifications:

American Board of Psychiatry and Neurology

American Board of Internal Medicine

American Board of Pediatrics

I Invest in Positive, Let it Flow into Your Life